LIVING WITH IT

Ways To Cope With Chronic Illnesses and Handicaps

Elizabeth Parsons Kirchner, Ph.D.

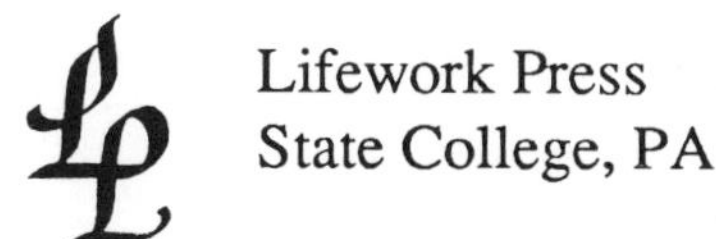

Lifework Press
State College, PA

Library of Congress Cataloging-in-Publication Data

Kirchner, Elizabeth Parsons, date.
   Living With It

   1. Chronically ill—Rehabilitation. 2. Handicapped—Rehabilitation.
3. Adjustment (Psychology) 4. Life skills I. Title
R108.K53 1988   649'.9   88-9460
ISBN 0-945404-02-6

CONTENTS

TO THE READER

I wrote this small book to pass along the wisdom of people who live well with difficult chronic conditions. Although I included some ideas from other writers, this book primarily offers what people with chronic conditions taught me in person. I often quote them anonymously. They are my friends, my relatives, and my clients (I am a clinical psychologist). My sisterly friend, Rana McMurray Arnold, and my sisterly cousin, Katharine Taylor Brennan, let me see most clearly what "living with it" really means. I dedicate this book to them.

I wish there were better terms than "chronic illness" or "permanent handicap" for conditions that won't go away. Other terms are prettier, but they don't call a spade a spade, and I want above all to be clear. If you are dealing with the challenges of a chronic illness or permanent handicap, you probably have enough confusion in your life. I also strive to be brief, so I often use "illness," "handicap," and "condition" interchangeably.

While some things in this book may not be in harmony with your special situation, I hope much will be compatibly useful to you. Please glean what fits and disregard the rest. You will add your own wisdom as you go along.

$$1.$$

WHAT IS "CHRONIC," ANYWAY?

When you have a chronic illness, disability, or condition, you are not acutely sick, although you may be from time to time. You aren't totally ill, but you aren't totally well either. You aren't totally handicapped, but you aren't totally able-bodied.

Some Similarities Among Chronic Conditions

Chronic conditions have these characteristics in common:

- They don't go away. They are permanent.
- They involve treatment that doesn't cure, but aims to control symptoms and long-range effects.
- They interfere with many normal activities and routines.
- They take time and limit your energy.
- They frequently strain financial resources.
- They require you to modify your life goals, vocational path, and recreational pleasures.
- They bring changes in friendship and family roles.

Psychologically, chronic conditions are similar in these ways:

- They threaten your self-esteem and your sense that you are the master of your own body.
- They are full of uncertainty.

- They upset your sense of being able to handle things.
- They involve fear that significant people will withdraw, and that you will lose love, approval, and support.
- They involve fear of strangers providing care and in-
  truding into your life and decisions.
- They involve fear of pain, injury, and loss of body
  parts.
- They confront you with your own mortality.
- They bring you face-to-face with the fact that much as
  you would like to believe that life is fair, it isn't.

Some Differences Among Chronic Conditions

Although chronic illnesses and conditions have a lot in common, there are big differences among them that determine what
you have to deal with.

Maybe you have something that doesn't show. In that
case, you look well on the outside when you don't feel
that way on the inside.

...Or...

Maybe your condition is visible to other people. You
may not look okay on the outside, even when you feel
okay.

Maybe your difficulty came on gradually.

...Or...

Maybe it happened suddenly, traumatically.

Maybe it's getting steadily worse.

...Or...

Maybe it has its ups and downs or has periods of re-
mission.

Maybe it is fatal or life-threatening.

...Or...

Maybe it isn't.

Whatever your specific difficulty, you will live with it the rest of your life. You join increasing numbers of people living with chronic conditions. You are not alone.

You Are Not Alone, But You Are Unique

It can be tremendously comforting to know you are not alone. But at the same time, you are not the same as anyone else. How you live with your condition, how you accommodate your life and your spirit to your situation, is going to be related to:

- What kind of person you are: your traits, values, and beliefs.
- What you have learned up until now about adapting to difficult situations, and how creative you are.
- Your life-stage; whether you are a child, adolescent, young adult, mid-life adult, or older adult.
- Your life-style; whether you are living alone or with your parents, spouse, friend, lover, or adult children; whether your family is large or small.
- Whether your financial picture is bleak, adequate, or bountiful.
- Your occupation and interests.
- The options and limitations of your housing and your community.
- Your friendships and emotional support network.

Because you are unique in your coping style, life situation, and illness, not everything in this book will apply to you.

Does Any of This Fit?

The experiences listed below are normal for people living with chronic illness. You may face only some of these challenges. Others you may meet only at certain times. You will no doubt find you can add some of your own.

- You never expected anything like this to happen to you.
- You want it to go away.
- You wish just trying harder would make it go away.
- You want everything medical science has to offer, but you wish some medical procedures were not so frightening, impersonal, and painful.
- You want to be told everything, but you dread knowing.
- You feel helpless and hopeless at times.
- You must make important decisions without enough information.
- You are afraid decisions will be made behind your back.
- You don't want to worry other people but you do want their love and concern.
- You hold back because you don't want to be a complainer.
- You don't want people to reject you, leave you, or hurt you.
- You are afraid of loneliness. Still, sometimes you just want to be left alone.
- You feel like a bundle of contradictions.
- Your illness makes you feel inadequate and undesirable.
- It's a battle to keep up your self-esteem.
- You could use a little more understanding.

— You could use a little less uncertainty.
— Sometimes you just want a hand to hold.
— Sometimes you just want to give up.
— You can't stand pity.
— You don't like self-pity either, but you feel it at times.
— You've had enough suffering.
— You've had enough loss.
— You want a vacation from it all.
— You often think "if only . . . ."
— You don't sleep, play, or concentrate well.
— Your condition crowds out thinking about other things.
— You're low on energy, motivation, and hope.
— You want a cure.

Remember that no matter what difficulties, limitations, and uncertainties your condition imposes, you also have similar goals to those of a well person. These goals are to live your life as fully as possible and to function as well as possible in all aspects of your life. Coming to live well with chronic conditions means fitting a new reality to these goals.

2.

FACING IT

One of the lessons you are sure to learn when you live with a chronic condition is that there is room in the scheme of things even for the unexpected, the unfair, and the tragic. You come to grips with what has occurred simply because it has occurred.

An author unknown to me expressed the reality of living with something-that-is-here-to-stay this way:

> *You just have to say it;*
> *That's the way it is.*
> *It's that way because*
> *It's that way.*

Although you never expected to have to come to terms with a chronic illness, it helps to know that it is a common lifetime experience; it is a process that can be dealt with.

The specifics of adaptation are different for everyone. The basics are pretty much the same for everyone.

3.

THE BASICS OF COMING TO LIVE WITH IT

In a simple way of looking at it, coming to grips with chronic illness involves these stages:

1. An initial period of shock and denial.
2. A time of restructuring and adjustment that involves depression, anger, grief, and anxieties.
3. A final stage of accommodation.

There are flaws in this oversimplified view. A more complete picture includes these points:

- You won't complete one so-called stage, proceed neatly to the next one, and then arrive, all tasks complete, at accommodation. You won't "succeed" or "fail," because adapting is a continuous process.
- You will re-experience all the issues of the adapting process often, sometimes in combination.
- Some people may be able to skip a grade in school, but no one can successfully skip any aspect of the adapting process.
- At different times you will deal with the issues of living with your condition at different levels of meaning and usefulness.

- Your progression will not be in a straight line. It will be more like a line spiraling mostly upward, with ups and downs along the way.
- The drain on your adaptive energies will be light at times and profound at others.
- People close to you — your family and close friends — will experience this process, too.

4.

DENIAL

Oh No!
It's not true. It can't be true.
It will all go away.
I don't have what they say I have.
I don't believe it.

When I was coming out of anesthesia for cancer surgery I told everyone present that I didn't need surgery, that I hadn't had any operation and that I was now in my own living room. Later, when my surgeon was discussing various oncologists (cancer specialists) he might refer me to, I kept thinking, "What on earth would I need an oncologist for?" These are just two personal examples of denial.

It is good that no one can escape initial denial. It is nature's way of helping us adjust to threat. This "ostrich reaction" helps us get through frightening and threatening times. It is the most common and most immediate way we deal with anxiety.

It is possible to maintain a stance of denial forever, but it cannot be done well. Merciful as denial is at first, if it goes on too long, it can keep you from taking an active part in adapting to the realities of your situation. In adapting, denial gradually gives way to acknowledging the condition.

5.

WHY ME?

There really is no answer to this question, but it keeps coming up.

Why me?

Did I do something wrong? Am I a bad person? Did I do something I shouldn't have done? Does God have it in for me?

Did I somehow want to punish myself? Should I have taken better care of myself? Should I have gone for treatment sooner? Did I bring on my own punishment?

> *Well, I know I have done some things wrong. Yes, I am guilty of some mistakes. And sometimes I do punish myself. But even if I think that I am being punished or that I am punishing myself, I can decide when I've had enough of that belief.*

Why me?

Because I could bear this burden better than someone else?

> *Well, I'm having some success dealing with it, but I'd rather have used my talents elsewhere.*

Why me?

Was this just bad luck . . . the luck of the draw as card players call it?

Maybe that's all there is to it.

Still . . . *why me?*

6.

ANGER

Asking "Why me?" is a natural reaction to bad news and to being treated unfairly. So is anger. Often intense anger surprises and puzzles you because you don't know where to direct it. To people around you? To God? To the medical people? To yourself? To anyone at all who is there at the wrong time?

Sometimes, for no reason at all, you blow up at someone for some simple thing. It's all out of proportion. You just fall apart and lose control. But it's *not* for no reason at all. Two reasons are:

- Behind anger is hurt. Being chronically ill means you have been hurt emotionally.
- Behind anger is frustration. Being chronically ill is chronically frustrating.

You feel awful about your outbursts and there are apologies to be made, but it helps to go easy on yourself. You will turn people away if you act chronically angry and it's better for everyone when you don't let anger accumulate, yet you don't always succeed. Know that when your frustrations pile up, you'll blow up.

And that it's natural.

And it beats growing bitter.

Not only is anger a natural feeling, it often leads to good out-comes. It can provide you the steam to stand up for yourself and take new actions on your own behalf.

When you express anger, it's best if you do it assertively (ex-pressing your feelings, needs, wants, and ideas without hurting someone else) and not aggressively (hurting someone in the process), although both will get you attention. It's worse if you are underassertive and don't stand up for yourself. Part of man-aging your chronic illness is not being "nice" all the time.

7.

DEPRESSION

Expect to get depressed. Everyone else does. You have more to be depressed about, just in case you need another reason.

Expect that when you are depressed, you will feel negative about yourself, about your situation, and about the future.

There may be days when:

- Nothing goes right.
- You don't care about anything.
- Tomorrow doesn't look any better.
- You feel like a failure.
- You don't want to see anyone.
- You cry a lot.
- You don't see any sense in going on.

It may help to know that:

- While depression doesn't feel good, it's normal.
- Life is a rollercoaster.
- It is okay to go under for a while.
- You don't have to do well all the time.
- Doing something really nice for yourself can help.
- New stimuli, ideas, and inputs can help.
- Anything to get your mind off how bad you feel can help.

You will learn about your own individual depression and the best ways to deal with it. You will learn by trial and error what it takes to get you through the night.

Adopt a functional approach. That means that if you find that something works for you, use it. If it doesn't work, don't use it. Most things don't work all the time, but you will find techniques that become your specialties for dealing with your times of depression.

If nothing seems to work for ordinary depression, remember:
The longest time it ever rained was 40 days and 40 nights and then the sun came out. The depression will lift.

For severe or unrelenting depression, remember:
It is something to get professional help with, because it can be alleviated.

8.

SOMETHING CAN ALWAYS BE DONE

One of the most devastating things a person can hear is, "There is nothing more I can do for you." The devastation comes if you think it means, "Nothing more can be done at all."

Until our last breath, something can always be done. Adapting over and over again to a condition that brings increasing difficulties can be incredibly hard. Yet it is possible to find things that can be done, even when your highest hopes have been dashed.

It may be true that a particular professional can do no more to help you. If he or she says, "There is nothing more I can do," you might want to ask, "Who or what *could* help? How do I get the information?"

A regular eye doctor, for example, may not be trained to help someone with severe sight-loss. But a low-vision specialist may have something to offer, and nonmedical avenues of help are always open. Even with total sight-loss, there are professionals, agencies, support groups, and individuals who can do many, many things in terms of aids, information, and training to help you keep adapting to your new situation.

The wisdom in "living with it" when "it" gets worse is to hold to the reality that there will always be something to make it possible and easier for you to live with its heartbreaks and adversities.

That "something" is often an increase in spirituality. For most people, a closer relationship to God and a greater reliance on religious and philosophical moorings are primary sources of help and sustenance. This book is an earthly and practical companion for you to take along on many religious and philosophical paths.

9.

EVERYDAY COPING

Living with chronic illness means you have a lot of coping to do.

Stress is inevitable whether or not chronic illness is in the picture. It comes as a result of changes that are part of each stage of life, sudden and serious events, and daily wear and tear. In addition to the stresses of the able-bodied, you will have extra stresses as a result of having a chronic condition.

You'll never be in total control, so don't try. Know that you don't have to be overwhelmed either, even though difficulties can sometimes pile up unmercifully. There is a middle path of dealing reasonably well and capably with the challenges in your life. The best overall advice I've ever found for dealing with stress tells us to separate what we have some control over from what we don't.

> *Grant me the serenity*
> *to accept the things I cannot change,*
> *the courage*
> *to change the things I can,*
> *and the wisdom*
> *to know the difference.* *

---

* These profound words, familiar to many people as the Serenity Prayer of Alcoholics Anonymous, are attributed to theologian Reinhold Neibuhr.

With stresses you have some control over, try this checklist. *

1. *Accept responsibility.* It's your life, and no one can cope for you. Other people can help, but the initiative and responsibility must come from you.

2. *Try to be objective.* Step back. Look at your situation as if it were someone else's. What could that person do? What would that person have to accept?

3. *Know your strengths and weaknesses.* Be honest with yourself; you need a clear picture of what you are working with.

4. *Don't try to cope alone.* Be ready to turn to family, friends and colleagues. Be ready to get outside help.

5. *Take a positive approach.* A solution may not be immediately apparent or easy, but you can find one or more things to try. It will always be possible to do *something*.

6. *Be realistic.* Don't expect too much of yourself. Some things you can solve only indirectly or partially. Set attainable goals.

7. *Don't strain for absolute control.* You'll just waste time and effort. Sometimes your only possible way to cope will be to withdraw from the situation, relax, and put it out of mind for a while.

---

* Adapted with permission of the Canadian Mental Health Association from its publication, *Coping with Everyday Problems.*

8. *Relax. Get pleasure.* Things that relax you and give you pleasure are nourishment and give you energy at any time. Use them whether or not you are having difficulty.

9. *Be flexible.* If your first idea doesn't work, try something else. Mistakes give you information for the next try. And it is the fact that you acted — took charge — that counts.

10. *Take one step at a time.* Several problems at once? Pick the easiest one first. Find the first small step to deal with it. Then do it. Work on the rest in easy stages. Write things down if that helps you take one step at a time.

11. *Put your sense of humor to use.* Look for something in the problem to laugh at. Humor brings relief and, perhaps, a new perspective.

12. *Reward yourself along the way.* It can be hard work. You deserve a prize.

All conditions that don't go away involve both general coping strategies and specific ones to deal with the limitations your particular condition brings. It can seem you're always experimenting . . . and you are! It may help to remember that:

• Experts are amateurs in situations that are new to them. If your condition changes, some previously successful strategies may no longer work, and you may start as an amateur again until you find new strategies that do work.

- Even with no particular changes in your condition, a strategy may work one time and not the next. It may work again next week.
- Something that works well in one situation may work poorly or not at all in another situation.
- It's generally smart to give strategies a good try, but you don't have to try harder and harder. You can go easy on yourself. A balance between active striving and passive letting-it-be is possible.

10.

SOME OTHER THINGS TO TRY

As you shift to new ways of doing things, you keep investigating what works best for you. Here are some additional approaches to consider in case you aren't already acquainted with them. They help many people, but only your personal experience will say whether they work for you.

Techniques to Control Tension, Conserve and Mobilize Energy, and Create Inner Calm

If there were one sure-fire technique that worked for everyone, there wouldn't be so many possibilities for you to consider.

A few advocates claim everyone can be helped by a particular approach. Don't believe them. On the other hand, you don't have to be put off by their extravagant claims if you want to find out if that approach helps you.

Among these potentially helpful resources are biofeedback, hypnosis, desensitization, and imagery. They usually require a professional to personally train you.

Other possibly powerful resources are relaxation and meditation techniques. One-on-one is a common way to learn them, but you can also explore their benefits through group classes, books, articles, and TV programs.

Several brands of all the approaches are available. Some are plain and simple. Others are more elaborate. Some involve a particular belief system or philosophy. Even if you already have your own good methods for dealing with tension, energy loss, and overload, trying a programmatic approach may extend your skills considerably.

Good Fun and Laughter

One of the most serious things I can ask is that you insist on having good fun and laughter. They are life-promoting, health-promoting, and essential for your sanity.

I don't mean putting on an up-beat front, acting cheerful, or trying to be funny yourself. Those efforts are well worth making, but here I mean something else. I mean getting the boost that is provided to you by your fondest sources of fun and laughter. You don't have to create the humor. It is there for you.

Get grins, belly-laughs, silliness, chuckles, giggles, snickers, and roars from your favorite sources of sheer entertainment of the humorous kind. A few possibilities are TV comedies, circuses, song-fests, joke books, funny movies, and funny people.

It isn't just a marvelous distraction that you get from a deliberate regimen of humor. You also get an increase in your body's natural chemicals that fight infection and depression.

A Personal Journal

A personal journal is usually more than — and different from — a daily diary, although you might also want to keep a record of daily happenings. A personal journal is a way to:

- Express privately the things you can't tell anyone else.
- Get your ideas "out there," to clarify your thoughts and feelings.
- Free your insights.
- Keep descriptions of important people and events.
- Focus on a topic and look for new perspectives.
- Profit from solitude.

There are no rules to follow. You can write in any way that suits your purposes of the moment. You don't have to use sentences or paragraphs. You could try lists. Or letters-you-know-you'll-never-send. Or conversations with yourself. You could use a journal-book, a regular tablet, or scraps of paper. You don't even have to write; you can use a tape recorder.

The relief and clarifications of journal-keeping are immediate benefits. There will be benefits later, too, if you save what you have written or recorded. You will be able to look back on your previous experiences and see how you saw things then. You will discover your process of adapting. It will reaffirm that, as you meet the challenges of living with something that won't go away, your central relationship is with yourself.

11.

ADVICE FOR EMERGENCIES: FIRST, FLY THE PLANE

Ordinary coping isn't enough in emergencies. When everything seems out of control, getting to the basics of keeping yourself functioning is the number one priority so you can deal with the crisis.

A pilot I know was taught to memorize this simple prescription to use in emergencies:

First, Fly the Plane

and then remember the Four C's:

Communicate
Confess
Conform
Climb

What if you were a pilot and became utterly lost, or discovered some equipment failure, or saw everything in the plane starting to come loose and go out the window? The single most important thing you could remember to do first would be just to keep the plane flying. You would disregard everything not related to helping the plane to fly . . . which, incidentally, it was built to do. Then you would use the Four C's.

Now for the Four C's:

- *Communicate* means that when you are in trouble you get in touch with someone who can understand you and your situation. Immediately.

- *Confess* means that you state your situation clearly and briefly. Don't beat around the bush. Don't apologize or make excuses. Don't worry about saving face.

- *Conform* means you take advice. Don't argue.

- *Climb* means you gain altitude and get above the clouds so you can see better and coast longer while you decide what to do next.

You may want to adapt this prescription to "fly the plane and use the Four C's" for personal crises and emergencies. The first priority is focusing on the basics of keeping yourself functioning . . . real basics like breathing well, staying warm, drinking enough fluids, and getting enough rest and good nourishment. Then you can deal with the crisis by communicating, confessing, conforming, and climbing. It could keep you from crashing.

12.

EXPECT GROWTH

N ot all stress is bad for you. Although your character and spirit will be sorely tried at times, coping well with challenges means you advance in personal development. All the adapting you do means you acquire wisdom others may never achieve.

If people went along with no stresses at all — a situation admittedly absurd to contemplate — they would simply not grow and develop. Because you are dealing with larger-than-average stresses, there is the likelihood that you will grow in ways you might not otherwise have thought you could.

ON BEING WONDERFUL

I think I'm supposed to be an inspiration to others. Is that my real purpose? I feel the expectation in others' eyes.

When people see you at your best, they see you accomplishing what they think they couldn't manage if they were in your shoes. In admiration and even awe, they may say to you, "I don't know how you do it." And to others they may say, "Isn't he (or she) wonderful!"

What they may not see is that you would prefer not to have to deal with your condition at all. You aren't always "wonderful," and you don't like having always to be "wonderful." They don't see that it isn't easy for you, any more than it would be for them. Yet you are doing it, because, well, you can't choose not to have your illness.

That's where your being an inspiration comes in. People admire you for adapting to a condition that, given the choice, everyone would prefer not to be living with. And perhaps they know other people in situations similar to yours who are not managing as well as you are.

What can you do if you hear how wonderful you are and feel both proud and uncomfortable at the same time?

You can:

1. Take the credit. You earned it.

and...

2. Let at least some people know it isn't possible always to be wonderful.

and...

3. Let yourself know it's crazy to try always to meet other people's expectations that you will be wonderful. The burden of upholding an image adds too much to the load you already carry.

14.

MINOR MIRACLES

Extraordinary things can happen when you least expect them.

Yesterday my spirit was badly bruised. Nothing seemed to be going well. From out of nowhere, this stranger leaned down to me in my wheelchair and whispered, "Don't despair."

I couldn't sleep and I looked out on the lights of the city. I had seen it all before, but this time I had a great sense of wonder about all of life and how powerful human intelligence is to put all that together. It was tremendously comforting to know I was a part of it all.

They were just ordinary sea shells, lying on the window sill. The sun shone on them and suddenly they looked incredibly beautiful, like a work of art. Amazing, the lift I got out of that.

I picked up one of those old magazines that are always in waiting rooms. It practically opened itself to an article on a problem we were having. It was like an answer to a prayer.

There may be better explanations for these wonderful experiences, but I like to call them minor miracles. Be receptive to the mystery in everyday life. Welcome the unexpected meanings in ordinary happenings and those unexplainable but uplifting events.

As the saying goes:

Don't just believe in miracles, *rely* on them.

15.

REACHING OUT

I've learned a lot in the last three years. I've learned mostly that I can't do everything myself. I've learned that it's really one of the most important things in life to be able to reach out when you need to. I always played "the strong one." It was the thing that was hardest for me to learn or to do, to reach out to other people. Yet when I do reach out to them they're very accepting and they respond in such a way that I know it makes them feel good because I think people really do want to give. They want to feel that they are necessary, that they are involved in your life.

I have examples of that all around me. I have all these cards people have sent me, and flowers, and phone calls, and just good wishes. And there are people like a friend's mother who lights a candle for me in her church, and people who pray for me, people whom I've never met but know about me through my friends and relatives.

People want to help.

Part of managing chronic conditions is marshaling your "people resources" by reaching out to them.

Here are two examples:

- A woman whose leg has been amputated keeps a list of things she needs help with, places she can't get to alone, and things she would enjoy doing with someone else. When someone says "Let me know if there's anything I can do," she selects a few items appropriate for that person and says, "Well, some things on my list are A, B, C, and, D. Would you like to do any of those?" When you can be specific, the other person doesn't have to guess, perhaps incorrectly, what you would truly enjoy or find helpful.

- A man with sight-loss found that the friends who usually read to him were becoming less available for one reason or other, so he advertised in the newspaper for volunteer readers. He not only found new readers but some new friends as well.

Not everyone responds the way you might hope when you reach out to them. But most certainly you will forsake much of what you need if you don't let someone know you need it.

I know there is a danger that some people "use" their handicap — they ask for more than they need and avoid responsibility for doing things they are perfectly able to do for themselves. It is a danger to avoid. But it is a small one compared with the danger that you will put off learning to reach out to people as an effective way to adapt to your illness.

16.

FRIENDS

At various times in your life you need good luck, good food, good doctors, and good escapes, but the one thing you need all your life is a good friend.

It is important to have different friends for different needs. People who have different backgrounds and experiences have much to give to each other and much to learn from each other. It is a good idea to have at least one friend who is:

- Older
- Younger
- Richer
- Poorer
- Smarter
- Dumber

Whether you prefer a small or large group of friends, you need at least one good friend with whom you feel easy rapport and to whom you can confide anything you want to — someone who will "be there" for you emotionally.

Even with old friends, you often have to take the first steps to talk about your condition. It is sad when misconceptions and fears about talking about it mean that both you and your friend go to great lengths to avoid the very topic that is probably uppermost in both your minds. You are the one who can best break through any barriers simply by speaking about your situation first.

Friendships change for everyone, whether chronic illness is in the picture or not. Some grow, some stay on the same level, some wither away. Most go through peaks and valleys. With chronic illness there are more challenges to friendship. Some friends disappoint you, some disappear, some become closer. Count on a few surprises.

Chronic illness can change the routines you cherish in your friendships. Because of your limitations, you may be unable to do some of the things you used to do with your friends (or you can do them less well or less often). The challenge is to come up with new and satisfying ways to both accommodate your restrictions and keep friendships. Home entertainment instead of active sports, perhaps, or more telephone visits and fewer business lunches, or some entirely new interest to take up together. Sometimes it isn't possible to find the right things to continue a friendship, and it simply can't be helped.

Because some old friendships will fade, keep building a reservoir of new acquaintances from which new friendships may grow. Friends ripen slowly, and they begin not as friends, but as acquaintances.

17.

STAYING VALUABLE
TO OTHERS

One trap in chronic illness is that you can be on the receiving end more than is good for you or your relationships. You can overlook the fact that it is *mutual* giving and receiving that builds and bonds relationships.

A hazard is that you can become absorbed in your situation. You can lose sight of balancing the give and take in a relationship. In a well-balanced relationship, each person needs something and has something special to give.

When you are on the receiving end too long and you overlook what you can give, the relationship can become unbalanced and weakened. People may stay with you, but it will be more out of obligation, pity, duty, or sainthood, all of which are poor grounds for a healthy relationship.

Another reason to balance receiving from others by giving to others is that it makes you feel good about yourself. You eliminate some of the self-esteem challenges that come with chronic illness when you know that even if your health is not normal, your relationships are.

What can you give? It doesn't depend on the amount of money, time, or energy you have. Three things — interest in the other person, thanks, and (sometimes) tokens of love and appreciation — are wonderfully ample to stay valuable to others.

1. First and always, give your interest in the other person. If you focus too much on your situation, even when people are genuinely interested, they will get B-O-R-E-D or otherwise uncomfortable, whether they show it or not. One likely result is that they will contact you less often, or for shorter times, or with less enthusiasm.

   There are graces I call "How's your job?/How's your dog?" questions. Be prepared to ask them. Listen with interest. Remember something important in the other person's life from your last contact with the person (this can take practice) and ask about that.

2. Always give thanks. Use your own style. The only style that doesn't work is assuming the other person knows you appreciate something. Even if you both are mind readers, say thank you in person, in writing, or in things you give.

3. Sometimes, give things. Tokens of your love and appreciation can be anything you make, buy, or find. It is the thought that counts. The most precious thing I ever received was a stack of small plastic supply jars collected for me by someone who had been isolated in a hospital room for two months.

18.

YOUR CLOSEST RELATIONSHIPS

When you live as part of a couple or family and a chronic condition enters the picture, everyone's life is affected. In different degrees each person will experience the challenge and strain of the adaptation process — denial, depression, anger, and coming to terms with your condition.

Each person's behavior patterns and personal development will be altered from the usual or "normal" ones that apply when everyone is able-bodied. Everyone's task will be to adapt to the condition for what it is, not magnifying or minimizing the effects.

Sad but true, because of the added stresses for everyone involved, chronic illness has the potential to magnify any long-standing difficulties in a relationship. As a countermeasure it usually helps for everyone to have — or to rapidly develop — clear ways of telling what their situation is and what they need and feel.

It also often helps to be able to talk more intimately. With open and free discussion, your relationships may grow closer and some previously unexpressed feelings and qualities in a person can be seen.

This is a good example of being able to share your feelings and clear the air with someone you love. It can help the other person do the same thing. It is a good example, too, of a common issue for handicapped people — irrational guilt.

With any of the people who are closest to you, you will sometimes feel guilty for having your illness, for "causing" them problems, for "putting them through all this." You regret that when you need to concentrate on your own health with its limitations and responsibilities, the people close to you also have limitations and responsibilities they ordinarily wouldn't encounter either.

Rationally you know you never elected to have your condition, and you should never seriously feel you have to apologize for the changes it demands. But every now and then you feel guilty. Feelings are facts, as they say. It's a good idea to share them, crazy or not, but don't go around apologizing all the time. You are not guilty.

What should you tell the people closest to you about your illness? It depends:

1. It is almost always best to tell your spouse or partner and any adolescent and adult children exactly

what your condition is, your predictions about it, and any significant changes you experience. You don't like surprises yourself, so don't withhold information, whether out of kindness or martyrdom. (Indeed, families do not like martyrs and do not treat them as well as they treat up-front people.)

2. Regarding elderly relatives, you naturally have to adapt what you tell them to their situation. Usually, though, anyone can take the truth better than fiction or secrecy.

3. Tell younger children the general picture and make sure they have you and others to answer their questions when they come up, which all parents know is when you least expect them. Don't be surprised if teenagers ask few questions or appear to be trying to ignore the whole matter.

Most of all, whether children or adults, the people closest to you need reassurances of your love. They need confidence that you will keep up your end of the relationship as much as possible. They need to know that although you cannot do some things, you can look for alternative routines and activities that are fully satisfying. They need to know that while you may have to give up some things and get help with other things, you are still very much their parent, partner, spouse, grown child, brother or sister, and so forth.

You can't give anyone anything better than a model of a person living well in your relationships in spite of chronic illness.

19

PROBLEM PEOPLE

People can be your most precious blessings. They can also give you your most exasperating moments.

Even the best-hearted of people can be "Problem People" who unwittingly react to chronically ill or physically limited people in ways that are as irritating as they are uninformed.

They may:

- Treat you as less mature and less capable than you are.
- Act toward you in patronizing or condescending ways.
- Act as though you are fragile when you aren't.
- Seem awkward and not genuine.
- Not give you accurate feedback, especially negative feedback.
- Give you exaggerated positive feedback.
- Step in to help without asking.
- Talk about you in your presence as though you weren't there.
- Talk excessively about *their* illnesses and problems.
- Talk too much about someone else who has a condition "just like yours."
- Say "I know exactly how you feel" when they haven't the slightest idea how you feel.

Besides these mistakes of conduct, Problem People show lamentable attitudes as well. For example:

- They may misinterpret a symptom for something else (if you have balance problems, someone could mistakenly think you are drunk).
- They may expect you to be bitter or stoic or something else, depending on how they think *they* might react.
- They may expect you to get better even when they "know" your condition is chronic.
- They may not expect as much from you as they could.
- They may expect you to be satisfied with or grateful for less than a well person.
- They may think that because you've lost some physical skills, you've lost social skills as well.

What should you do? Do you have to correct every potentially demoralizing act and misconception? By no means.

Problem People can usually learn better ways, but take on the job of teaching them only if it seems worth your while. There is a lot of thoughtlessness and stupidity about chronic conditions in the world; don't burden yourself with it all.

Let much of it just go by you. It is, after all, the other person's problem and not yours, unless you let it get to you. Save most of your energies for positive people.

If you choose to clear up misconceptions, use plain and informative replies. For some Problem People, you may be their first teacher about chronic conditions and they may be fast learners. Develop some good one-liners for common irritations.

The real hazard when Problem People treat you in their uninformed and unkind ways is that you can be swayed in nonconstructive directions:

- Your self-esteem and self-confidence can suffer.
- You may psychologically isolate yourself.
- You may become too passive and dependent.
- You may not stand up for your rights, wants, and opinions.

Remember that in spite of Problem People's attitudes and actions, you are a competent, responsible person whose chronic condition does not diminish your status or rights as an individual.

Remember that one of the benefits of adapting to your condition as a fact of your life and getting on with it is that Problem People don't erase your self-confidence. As a friend explained it, "The more you accept it yourself, the more other people get over your situation and deal with you normally."

20

HELPFUL PEOPLE

S ome people are Problem People. Other people can be just the right thing at the right time.

Usually, helpful people are your friends and your kin. Sometimes the helpful person is a professional counselor, psychologist, psychiatrist, or member of the clergy whose training and personality are a good match with your needs. The people I describe in this chapter are not professionals in the strict meaning of the word. They are, however, expert at what they do, which is what matters. They are support groups, personal panels, and companion advocates.

Support Groups

Support groups (also called self-help groups) have mushroomed in the last several years for good reasons. There may be one near you or you may want to start one.

Even if you don't feel like dealing with a group of people, you might want to ask to meet individually with someone from the group.

Effective support groups let you:
- Learn that you are not alone.
- Meet people who have gone through what you are going through.

- Get things off your chest.
- Feel understood and valuable.
- Add to your circle of supportive people.
- See how others have solved problems similar to
  yours.
- Share what's going on in your life.
- Talk about things you ordinarily wouldn't tell other
  people.
- Have a good time.

That last point is important. Effective support groups are living proof of positive adapting, and they make you feel good.

Personal Panels

I don't know anyone who has tried this idea in a difficult time during chronic illness, but I pass it along because it worked well for a young couple in another tough situation. Soon after their house and possessions were destroyed by fire, they asked a number of people they knew to be members of their "panel" to help them deal with the immediate and long-range issues they faced.

This small group — a few close friends, an insurance person, a financial/legal person, and a real estate person — met to put their heads together with the couple. Using the panel approach meant that the couple could get information and advice from several sources quickly and simultaneously. And it meant they were offered points to consider which they otherwise might have missed in their confusion and emotional overload.

Companion Advocates

I have used this idea myself and I swear by it. A companion advocate accompanies you through the maze when you are dealing with difficult medical decisions or procedures. A companion advocate can be with you at the doctor's office, the hospital, or any other place where you want someone with good memory, good knowledge, and good rapport with you and other people.

Especially when you must come to a decision promptly and are in shock or in pain, it can be tremendously helpful to have the "extra brain" of a companion advocate to help you handle a lot of information, remember details and ask the right questions. You may also feel the balm of the steady hand of this trusted person.

This person can be a family member, a friend, or anyone else you trust. Sometimes the apparently logical person may not be the right person. What you want is someone who, while at your side and on your side, can be calm, positive, and reasonably objective. You definitely need someone who is knowledgeable about the medical world and is neither intimidated by it nor antagonistic toward medical professionals.

Not everyone is able to find a companion advocate, but trained "patient representatives" or "patient advocates" have recently emerged as professional staff members at hospitals and other treatment facilities. They are there to explain the system, help you over the snags, and negotiate on your behalf.

21.

YOU AND YOUR PROFESSIONALS

When you have a chronic condition, you are sure to affiliate with an extensive cast of health care professionals. As in a long-running TV series, there are main characters, supporting cast, and bit players. Different players come on stage at different times in the series. All are important.

The Main Professional Characters

In the drama of chronic conditions, the main professional characters are your physicians. You and your primary physician play the leading roles. Other medical experts and specialists will play major roles from time to time.

Some points about doctors:

1. With any doctor, it is crucial that you have someone whose competence and judgment you trust. Why? Because if you don't have that trust, you won't be able to do your part in the alliance with your doctor, which is following his or her prescriptions for medication, other therapies, diet, and activities.

2. Most people find it is very important to like their primary physician in addition to having confidence in him or her. Liking seems less important with other physicians.

3. Wanting to help people directly is a strong reason doctors became doctors in the first place instead of, for example, research chemists. Beyond that similarity, they come in all flavors from vain and aloof to visibly compassionate and warm.

   Some of the technically best medical people may not react with the rapport or involvement you would prefer. If some doctors seem impersonal or grouchy, don't take it personally. Remember, they see many people with situations as bad or worse than yours every single day. They also have bad days like the rest of us.

4. It is pointless to keep shopping around for doctors, but you should always be willing to see another doctor for a second opinion when it is appropriate or to try another doctor if you are dissatisfied with one you have.

5. It helps if you can develop a workable way to let a doctor know when something is a true emergency or vitally important. Save everything else for your regular contacts.

Supporting Cast and Bit Players

Your supporting professional cast and bit players are any of the counselors, clergy, social workers, dieticians, nursing personnel, legal and government people, laboratory staff, and financial personnel who are involved in your situation.

You never know until you experience it how powerful each one can be.

> • Sometimes it is a professional person with whom you have a sustained relationship that "makes all the difference." It may be the continuing contacts with your social worker or counselor, for example, that make it possible for you to manage through a particularly stressful time better than you could without that person.

> • Sometimes it is a professional person who is there at the right time. It may be a talented nurse who knows the medical system and your situation who helps you when your intuition tells you something isn't going right but you can't put your finger on what is wrong.

> • Sometimes it is a nonmedical professional who keeps the business end of things from adding to your stressload. It may be someone from the financial office who spares you worry and fury by designing understandable business forms. Or it may be someone who smooths your path when you need to get records from somewhere else. Or someone who straightens out a complicated and exasperating problem with your medical insurance.

Little things mean a lot, too. The good-natured banter of a laboratory worker, for example, can make the day go better. On the other hand, any of the players can inadvertently be the last straw for you.

After all I had been through yesterday, I blew up at Mary from the dietary department because the soup was cold. It was all out of proportion. It had nothing to do with her, of course.

Sometimes you need a number of supporting professionals all at once. You have a right to ask for them. Whether or not all can respond, one way to keep yourself appropriately assertive is to ask for what you need. During a time of both medical and family crisis, someone I particularly admire for meeting difficulties superbly was readmitted to the hospital saying, "I need to see my surgeon, chaplain, psychiatrist, and social worker. Today."

The Setting

You and the professionals in your life play your roles in "stage settings" that are, initially at least, not familiar to you. Hospitals and medical procedures can make you feel as if you are an actor walking onto a stage where everyone except you knows what the act is.

Unfamiliar medical procedures bring the anxieties of the unknown. Even simple procedures that are routine to medical people can be needlessly frightening if you haven't been told what to expect.

Most professionals do a good job of informing you. But some forget that, even if a procedure is commonplace for them, you might not know anything about it. To avoid being surprised, let the person know if a procedure is new for you and ask for as much information as you want.

You can also feel the awkwardness of being on an unfamiliar stage when you are in the hospital.

As in any foreign territory, you acclimate better if you create some "personal space" within it. And you can deal with unavoidable stresses when you have personally comforting things around you.

Put your own cards and pictures on the wall, perhaps, or use your own pillow or blanket. I once took my sleeping bag with me to the hospital. A friend who was faced with his first stay in a hospital brought far too many books to read, but they weren't only for reading. They were also his "security blanket" and they signified his identity and interests to the other actors on the stage.

If you aren't on a special diet, you may also want to join the ranks of people who ask to have some of their favorite food brought in to them. Pizza, ice cream, or soda — whatever you crave from the outside — offers nourishment to your spirit inside.

This "nesting," no matter how you do it, is important. You create some personal space, announce your individuality, and bring comfort into an uncomfortable time.

22.

YOU'RE THE EXPERT

As you come to grips with your permanent condition and all its ramifications, you may find — scary as it is at times — that you are becoming your own best expert. You depend on professionals and other people in your life for what they can do, but you grow to depend on yourself as the expert on your own personal and unique situation. You keep seeking and discovering what works for you and what is best for you.

After all, no one can know as thoroughly as you do:
- The ins and outs of your mind and body
- Your disappointments and successes
- Your limitations and goals
- Your fears and hopes

I wrote this brief and general book to pass along the expertise of many people. The parts that are useful to you will become your expertise. You will "write your own book."

You may also want to read further and more extensively. Two books I recommend are authored by people who did indeed write their own book. They are:

Pitzele, Sefra K. *We Are Not Alone: Learning to Live with Chronic Illness*. New York: Workman Publishing, 1986.

and

Register, Cheri. *Living with Chronic Illness: Days of Patience and Passion*. New York. The Free Press, 1987.

As you become your own expert and find what works for you, I would love any feedback you care to send me. I wonder what was right on target for you, what was off the mark, and what was missing that you would especially like to have seen. You can always reach me at:

Lifework Press
Box 535
State College, PA 16804

ABOUT THE AUTHOR

Elizabeth Parsons Kirchner, Ph. D., is a graduate of Cornell University and The Pennsylvania State University. She has had a private practice for over 20 years and has been a psychology faculty member at Penn State and The State University of New York at Buffalo. She has held staff or consultant positions at several general and psychiatric hospitals.

Married and the mother of three grown children, she loves canoeing and hiking, pottery and photography, gardening and birdwatching. Having published extensively in the research and professional literature, she now writes primarily for a wider audience.